It's Not
"Just"
a Heavy Period

It's Not "Just" a Heavy Period

THE MISCARRIAGE HANDBOOK

ELIZABETH PETRUCELLI

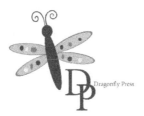

Dragonfly Press, LLC
Parker, CO

Published by:
Dragonfly Press, LLC
P.O. Box 161
Parker, CO 80134
Library of Congress Control Number: 2015933046
ISBN: 978-0-9851713-4-6
ISBN: 978-0-9851713-5-3 (eBook)

Edited by Amie McCracken
Cover Design by Elizabeth Petrucelli
Cover Image by freedigitalphotos.net (amenic181)

DISCLAIMER:

This book's aim is to serve as a guide for women. It is not intended to serve as medical advice. The author accepts no liability or responsibility for any loss or damage caused or thought to be caused by following the advice in this book and recommends that you consult a healthcare professional for medical advice or questions you may have with the advice contained herein.

For Ruby and Gus

Contents

ALSO BY ELIZABETH PETRUCELLI

All That is Seen and Unseen;
A Journey Through a First Trimester Miscarriage

The Miscarriage App
(available on Android and iOS)

Chapter One: It's Called Miscarriage But …

The term miscarriage is actually not a medical term even though we often hear it presented by care providers. Please note that the term abortion (used below) does not refer to medical or surgical abortions and only refers to "naturally occurring" death of the embryo/fetus. The terms used to define or describe miscarriage are:

- Spontaneous abortion / spontaneous miscarriage
- Complete abortion / complete miscarriage
- Incomplete abortion / incomplete miscarriage
- Missed abortion / missed miscarriage
- Inevitable abortion / inevitable miscarriage
- Threatened abortion / threatened miscarriage
- Blighted ovum
- Intrauterine fetal demise
- Live miscarriage
- Molar pregnancy
- Partial molar pregnancy
- Ectopic pregnancy

The last three are a different variation on pregnancy and pregnancy loss.

Terms you might hear to describe miscarriage:

- Chemical pregnancy
- There are no signs of you ever being pregnant
- No heartbeat
- No growth
- Baby stopped growing
- There is nothing there
- Not a viable pregnancy
- There is only a sac (blighted ovum)
- Pregnancy failure
- Embryonic demise

What the Baby Is Called

You may refer to your baby using the term baby; however, medically speaking you will likely hear these terms to refer to your baby.

- Embryo (conception to 11 weeks)
- Fetus (After 11 weeks)

Other terms used:

- Tissue
- Products of conception

Hearing these terms may be quite difficult for you. Medical staff don't typically use these terms to cause you any pain, they are only utilizing the terms assigned to them.

Definitions

A **miscarriage** is defined as a pregnancy loss prior to 20 weeks gestation. After 20 weeks gestation, the pregnancy loss is defined as a stillbirth. Miscarriage is the most common form of pregnancy loss and occurs in approximately one in four women.

A **spontaneous abortion** or **spontaneous miscarriage** occurs when the embryo or fetus is not viable, which means they are unable to survive, or when the embryo or fetus is born before 20 weeks gestation. It is usually just called "miscarriage."

A **complete abortion** or **complete miscarriage** occurs when the embryo and all products of conception (placenta, gestational sac) have emptied from the uterus. Cramping and bleeding typically subsides quickly following a complete miscarriage. An ultrasound is used to confirm.

An **incomplete abortion** or **incomplete miscarriage** occurs when only part of the embryo or fetus has emptied the uterus but other parts remain. Bleeding and cramping continue to occur although a woman may experience a decrease in cramping and bleeding, but after a period of time, the bleeding and cramping reoccurs and can be more intense.

A **missed abortion** or **missed miscarriage** occurs when the embryo dies but is not expelled from the uterus. Oftentimes, the mother discovers this during an ultrasound and no fetal heartbeat is detected for the proper gestational age or no further growth is seen when comparing previous ultrasounds.

An **inevitable abortion** or **inevitable miscarriage** occurs when there is dilation or effacement of the cervix and/or a rupture of the membranes (water breaks). It most commonly occurs with back pain and/or abdominal pain. These contractions cause the cervix to soften and open. If this continues, the embryo or fetus will be born.

A **threatened abortion** or **threatened miscarriage** occurs when there is vaginal bleeding accompanied with cramping but the cervix is not softening or opening. The woman may experience abdominal pain, lower back pain, and bleeding that is pink, brown, or red.

A **blighted ovum** occurs when the egg implants but no baby develops. There may be a yolk sac that develops inside the gestational sac but no baby forms. This can cause confusion on whether or not you were really pregnant. You were but there was a genetic problem that took place and the egg developed abnormally.

An **intrauterine fetal demise** occurs when a baby dies inside the uterus after 20 weeks gestation; however, some clinicians use this term for babies who die during pregnancy in the second trimester.

A **live miscarriage** occurs when the fetus is born and has a heartbeat. The baby may attempt to breath, may move and may survive for seconds, minutes, or hours, but no medical intervention can be performed due to how early the baby was born.

A **molar pregnancy** occurs in about 1 in 1000 pregnancies. It is also called a Hydatidiform mole which is a medical term meaning a fluid-filled mass of cells (mole = a mass of cells; hydatid = containing fluid-filled sacs or cysts). A molar pregnancy rarely involves a developing embryo and occurs due to a genetic error during fertilization. An ultrasound would reveal grape-like clusters with placental parts. Because a placenta forms, HCG is secreted and a positive pregnancy test can be seen. Unfortunately, there is no baby; only abnormal tissue grows and grows very rapidly in the uterus. A molar pregnancy is usually non-cancerous and is also referred to as gestational trophoblastic disease (GTD).

A **partial molar pregnancy** occurs when there are abnormal cells and a developing embryo. The embryo usually has severe defects and is quickly consumed by the abnormal tissue.

Molar and partial molar pregnancies require follow-up procedures /treatment and many doctors recommend waiting at least one year before attempting to conceive again (although this varies).

An **ectopic pregnancy** occurs when a fertilized egg implants outside the uterus. The most common location is implantation in the fallopian tubes, but an egg can implant in other locations although this is extremely rare. This is an extremely dangerous situation that can result in maternal death.

A **chemical pregnancy** occurs very early and results in bleeding around the time a woman would miss her period. Many women do not know they were pregnant and may notice heavier bleeding and cramping as well as possible clots and suspect pregnancy. A chemical pregnancy does not mean you weren't pregnant. It is a complication that occurs when a pregnancy is lost following implantation. HCG levels may rise enough to show a positive pregnancy test but shortly after the levels decrease due to the death of the baby.

Chapter Two: How It's Managed

There are three options for miscarriage: **expectant management, medical management and D&C (Dilatation and Curettage)**. These options are for confirmed miscarriage (baby no longer has a heartbeat or no growth) and blighted ovum. Believe it or not, this can be misdiagnosed and you could actually be performing a D&C on your living baby. It is imperative that vaginal (not abdominal) ultrasound be coupled with blood tests to ensure that your baby has, in fact, passed away before moving on to a D&C. Your care provider would note no visible heartbeat and falling HCG levels.

It is recommended that a minimum of two ultrasounds are performed on different days. Keep in mind that if you are very early in pregnancy (less than six weeks) your baby might not be detectable on an ultrasound (living or dead). HCG blood levels typically need to be above 1500mIU in order to see a gestational sac and/or fetal pole, and even then, the heartbeat might not be detectable until six weeks and three days or longer.

Waiting to find out is very difficult during this already stressful time, but this is the time where mistakes are most frequently made. Bleeding can be considered normal during very early pregnancy so bleeding alone is not a good indicator of an impending miscarriage. Bleeding coupled with cramping isn't even a good indicator, especially very early in pregnancy. It is recommended that you wait until at least seven weeks of pregnancy and have two ultrasounds to confirm pregnancy loss before proceeding to medical management or D&C.

These options are not for treating an ectopic pregnancy. Please consult your care provider if you believe you are experiencing a miscarriage. This information should not be substituted for medical advice.

Delivering naturally at home (expectant management of miscarriage): The risks are hemorrhaging (excessive bleeding), incomplete miscarriage (not all of the baby and placenta expelled) and infection. This option may lead to the need for an unplanned D&C (surgical treatment). It is important to monitor bleeding and watch for infection over the following weeks. You may experience moderate to intense pain. Your care provider can prescribe pain medications to help.

There is no research that explains when the miscarriage will start or how long it will take to complete. The miscarriage could begin shortly after diagnosis or take months to begin.

Using a medication to induce the miscarriage (medical management): The medication commonly used to induce miscarriage is Cytotec, also known as misoprostal. There are risks associated with taking this medication such as intense cramping and hemorrhaging. One benefit to using medication is timing of the miscarriage. The miscarriage will usually occur within a few hours after the first dose; although this varies greatly depending on gestational age of the baby. Sometimes utilizing this method can take several doses over several days and still lead to the need for surgical intervention. The medication can be taken sublingually, orally, or vaginally. It is most often given orally with early miscarriage and vaginally with second trimester miscarriage; although it can be administered either way.

There are side effects from the medication such as pain, cramping, nausea/vomiting, low grade fever and/or chills, skin rash and diarrhea. The risks are relatively the same as with a natural miscarriage: hemorrhaging, incomplete miscarriage and infection. Again, these could lead to needing a D&C. There are differing statistics on how effective this method is, with numbers ranging from 60%-90%.

Sometimes during hospital inductions for miscarriage, a foley bulb is used to help the cervix dilate. This is part of the induction process and may include the use of Pitocin — a synthetic hormone that stimulates uterine contractions. This may happen with babies who are between 16 and 20 weeks.

A D&C for miscarriage (short for dilatation and curettage), is an outpatient surgical procedure. This is most commonly performed in a hospital or a same-day surgery center, although some doctors are able to do this procedure in their office (reserved for very early miscarriages). Be sure that your doctor checks and then double checks that the baby has passed before choosing this option. Every baby's heartbeat starts at a different time. It is advisable to wait at least one week between ultrasounds to confirm the baby does not have a heartbeat, otherwise you may be aborting a viable fetus.

Most often you will be given a sedative and general anesthesia is used. Your legs are often placed in stirrups once on the operating table. This can feel awkward because your legs are placed there while you are still awake. If this process sounds like it may be uncomfortable for you, talk with the surgeon prior to the surgery.

The surgeon places a speculum in your vagina and begins to artificially dilate the cervix with instruments. They dilate the cervix just enough so that the vacuum can be inserted. The vacuum is also called "suction curettage" and scrapes the lining of the uterus and sucks out tissue.

The procedure usually takes anywhere from 15 to 30 minutes. It is rare that this procedure requires an overnight stay. You will also likely be given an antibiotic to prevent infection.

This procedure differs from a D&E (dilatation and evacuation) which is generally performed for miscarriages over 12 weeks gestation. The difference between the procedures is that during a D&E, the surgeon dilates the cervix and then uses a grasping instrument (forceps) to remove the baby (sometimes in parts) and then uses a vacuum to suction and scrape the remaining tissue in the uterus.

A D&C should be conducted with the use of an ultrasound to help guide the surgeon. Consult with your surgeon to ensure this is used. Failure to use the ultrasound can result in uterine perforation.

Risks Associated with the D&C:

- Adverse reaction to anesthesia medication
- Hemorrhage or heavy bleeding
- Infection in the uterus or other pelvic organs
- Perforation or puncture to the uterus
- Laceration or weakening of the cervix
- Scarring of the uterus or cervix (Asherman's Syndrome and can lead to infertility)
- Incomplete procedure which requires another procedure to be performed

The Benefits of a D&C Are:

- It can be scheduled
- Can provide enough tissue for testing (if you choose this)
- May bring closure or relief if you have been waiting for the inevitable miscarriage

If you want your baby intact, it is best to deliver at home or in the hospital with or without induction medication. Seeing your very early baby may be traumatizing. Always be sure you have someone with you while you are miscarrying. There are doulas who specialize in supporting families through loss. These doulas may be called Bereavement Doulas, Loss Doulas, or Baby Loss Family Advisors. A search on the internet should reveal a doula in your area.

If you deliver in a hospital, bonding time with baby should be encouraged. While at home, you will have as much time as you would like with your baby. If you are at home and need time to plan the final resting place for your baby, you may place your baby in your refrigerator.

Note:

If you are Rh negative and experience a miscarriage, you may need the Rh immunoglobulin injection. Please talk with your care provider. If your body produces antibodies due to the baby being Rh positive, this can cause serious complications during a later pregnancy.

Preventing Asherman's Syndrome

One of the best ways to prevent Asherman's Syndrome is to use medical management for your miscarriage. While it can be more painful, it can prevent future complications due to scar tissue. If you choose to have the D&C, it is highly recommended that your surgeon conduct an ultrasound-guided D&C instead of the normal blind D&C. Using the ultrasound while performing this procedure helps the surgeon to see where they need to use the suction instead of just blindly scraping inside of your womb and possibly damaging more areas. This also helps reduce the chances of needing a repeat procedure for failing to remove all the products of conception.

Following the procedure, your surgeon may place a balloon or stent inside your uterus for approximately two weeks. The balloon may also be referred to as a splint. This is not the standard of care; however, some surgeons utilize this technique. The splint is placed inside the uterus and a catheter runs out of your vagina which allows bleeding and fluids to come out. Placing this splint inside your uterus may help prevent the layers of the uterus from binding to each other causing the scar tissue known as Asherman's Syndrome.

Another therapy that may be utilized by your surgeon is estrogen therapy. This therapy may be combined with the splint therapy above. Estrogen therapy lasts for approximately 2 to 4 weeks and helps encourage healing by slowing progesterone production; thus slowing the building of the lining of the uterus while your uterus heals. There are risks to utilizing estrogen therapy such as blood clots so you will need to discuss the benefits versus the risks with your care provider.

Chapter Three: Options for Your Baby's Body

Bonding

Even the tiniest of babies, no matter where you birth your baby, can have many of these options.

- Cut the baby's cord.
- Preserve your baby's cord. A placenta encapsulator can help you dry your baby's tiny cord as a keepsake or consider an umbilical cord keepsake.
- Hold your baby (even if the baby only fits in the palm of your hand).
- Play music. Use music to imprint your brain and help you bond with your baby. Many women choose one song that is very meaningful to them. There is a list of songs in Chapter 12: Other Resources.
- Use essential oils. Create a specific blend of oils to diffuse in your room as you are holding and bonding with your baby.

- Take pictures with and of your baby. You may never want to look at them again, but knowing you have them available to view any time you want is very comforting.
- Have hand/footprints or hand/foot molds done by the hospital staff. Even tiny babies as early as 14 weeks can have their handprints and footprints taken by a skilled staff member.
- Bathe your baby. For small babies, sometimes holding them with you while you are in a tub of water can be very bonding and healing.
- Wrap the baby in a special blanket or outfit. Some hospitals can provide this but there are many organizations that make tiny outfits or special blankets for even the smallest of babies.
- Have your baby blessed or baptized.
- Name your baby.

Final Disposition for the Physical Form of Your Baby's Body

You have the right to choose the final arrangements of your baby's body regardless of gestational age. There are several options available with the most common options being **burial (communal or separate)**, **cremation (hospital incineration or private)** and **hospital disposition**.

Burial

The option for burial may be carried out in several different ways depending upon the wishes of the parents as well as state and local laws. In each case it is the responsibility of the parents to make the arrangements but oftentimes healthcare professionals and/or local funeral homes may assist with this process. Getting recommendations from friends and family can be helpful when making this decision. Sometimes it is too difficult to make this decision on your own. If it feels difficult for you, ask a family member or friend to make the calls for you.

Home

Sometimes, burying your baby at home is an option. You must check with your local county and state laws to see if this is an option for you. Sometimes this option is based on the size of the land or the location within city limits. Many people do not choose this option because of the possibility that they might move away from their home.

Cemetery

Purchasing a burial plot is another option. Some funeral homes are not attached to a cemetery but they will be able to list options for you on where your baby can be buried. You should talk with several funeral homes to find the best one to suit your needs and financial goals.

Some areas have communal burial plots where many babies are buried together. This is usually reserved for miscarriage as stillborn babies are not usually included in a communal burial. Some cemeteries may also allow your baby to be buried with another family member.

Cremation

The parents are responsible for choosing a funeral home for cremation of their baby's remains. You may choose to receive your baby's ashes or to ask if the funeral home disposes of them. Due to the small size of some babies, there may not be enough ashes to return to you.

Some crematories will release baby's ashes in a memorial garden. Talk with the crematory about the options you have. You may also desire to purchase an urn or cremation jewelry to store your baby's ashes. Sometimes, crematories will let you burn items with your baby such as letters or clothing but this policy will vary with each crematory. Please consult your religious leader as keeping your babies ashes may not fall in line with your church's teaching (for example, it is forbidden for Catholic's to scatter, divide, or keep their deceased loved ones ashes).

Hospital Disposition

Choosing this option usually means your baby will be incinerated in an approved medical incinerator. Your baby may or may not be incinerated with hospital/medical waste. Some hospitals incinerate babies separated from medical waste, but not all do this. If you are concerned about the final disposition of your baby's remains, this might not be the best option for you. Usually, the baby's remains cannot be returned to you. Some hospitals release the remains of babies in an area on hospital grounds, usually at a memorial site, that families can visit. Discuss this option with hospital personnel.

Final Note:

Many funeral homes and crematories offer their services for reduced rates and some even offer their services for free. Please check with your local funeral homes and crematories to see if this is offered there. Most will tell you upfront as a courtesy. In some areas, the coffin is also free although it is a basic coffin. Urns are usually not free.

Chapter Four:
Experiences

What You Might Experience

There is no single way to experience a miscarriage. Everyone's experience will be different. The most common description of a miscarriage is, "It's just a heavy period." While some women may experience miscarriage this way, the majority of women do not. Your miscarriage experience will also depend greatly on the gestational age of your baby.

A **chemical pregnancy** (extremely early pregnancy loss), may result in a heavier period. Most commonly, the woman reports she was a day or two "late" and had more clots, heavier bleeding and stronger cramping. Because a chemical pregnancy is lost so close to when a woman would usually start her period, many women don't even realize they were pregnant and suspect a pregnancy only due to how different this period was from others in her past.

From conception to week four: Women are discovering they are pregnant earlier now than any other time in history. Part of this is due to the technological advances in pregnancy tests which allow for early detection but another aspect is due to advances in assisted reproductive technology. This includes cycle monitoring, medications, artificial insemination, in-vitro fertilization and other fertility treatments. Women are testing earlier and announcing pregnancies earlier. It is now commonplace for a woman to announce her pregnancy as early as three to four weeks. This results in women knowing they are experiencing a pregnancy loss very early. Fifty percent of all pregnancy losses occur at this stage of pregnancy.

From weeks four to eight: women have reported their miscarriage as painful and much more than just a heavy period. Women experience heavy bleeding and cramping, large clots and the passing of gray tissue. Women have taken pictures of the tiny babies they have birthed although most women will only see gray tissue or tiny fragments of placenta. Once the heartbeat is seen, less than 5% of women miscarry at this stage of pregnancy.

From weeks eight to 13 (beginning of the second trimester): women have reported their miscarriage as similar to labor, having a contraction pattern that is intense with their pain ending at the birth of their baby. Some women report feeling their baby slide through their vagina and fall into the toilet, bath, or into their hands. Many of these babies are fully intact and some are still within their gestational sac.

From weeks 13 to 20: the experience of miscarriage is far from "just a heavy period." Women experience contractions and heavy bleeding. They often present in the emergency room and learn they are having a miscarriage. Some of their babies are born alive but too small and fragile for any life-saving medical intervention. The family can see and hold their baby. One to five percent of miscarriages occur at this stage of pregnancy.

Warning Signs

If you experience any of the below signs, please contact your care provider immediately or visit your closest emergency room.

- Increased vaginal bleeding which is not related to an increase in physical activity
- Vaginal bleeding that soaks more than one pad per hour
- Passing blood clots that are larger than a golf ball
- Fever over 100.3 degrees Fahrenheit
- Swollen, red, painful area on your leg (sign of a blood clot)
- Signs of vaginal or uterine infection: redness, swelling, pain and/or foul smelling drainage from vagina
- Pain or burning while urinating
- Inability to urinate
- Severe constipation that is not relieved by diet change or laxative use
- Intuition tells you something is wrong

Caring for Your Postpartum Body

Even though you didn't deliver a full term baby, the physical and emotional states are very much the same of a postpartum mother and you will need to care for your body in a similar way. Below is a list of things to help you care for your postpartum body.

- Take naps and try to get plenty of rest.
- Limit visitors unless visits are emotionally healing for you.
- Your bleeding will get lighter as the days progress but you may bleed for up to six weeks.
- Your bleeding may increase with too much activity. If you notice bright red blood or blood after you stopped bleeding, you may have engaged in too much physical activity. The placenta leaves a wound in your womb that needs time to heal. Exercise is very helpful but start slow and easy.
- Nothing should be placed in your vagina for six weeks. This includes sexual intercourse, tampons, items that strengthen the perineal muscles, fingers, or sexual toys. Introducing anything into the vagina increases your risk of infection.
- Lifting should be restricted to items less than 15 pounds.
- Household chores should be put on hold or completed by someone else for the first few weeks while your body heals.
- Eat healthy foods.
- Drink plenty of fluids (at least six to eight glasses of water per day)

- Change your pads every two to three hours. This will help reduce the risk of infection.
- If you received a peri-bottle, use this every time you urinate. (Some women with first trimester miscarriage will not receive this).
- If you have vaginal pain in your perineum, you can soak in a small amount of water in the bath tub. A hemorrhoid pillow can also be helpful and can be found at most drug stores.
- Increase your fiber intake to help with any constipation. Short walks every day will also help with moving your bowels and reduce constipation.
- Urinate every three to five hours to reduce the risk of contracting a bladder infection.
- Do not drive if you are taking any narcotics for pain.
- Avoid smoking, illegal drugs, alcohol and limit caffeine consumption.

What You Might Feel

Everyone feels different about miscarriage and pregnancy loss. There are no right or wrong reactions to miscarriage. It is just as normal to be devastated as it is normal not to grieve. Some believe they lost a baby or future child, while others believe they lost a ball of cells which had the potential to become a baby or child. No matter what you believe, you may still be very sad about this loss.

There is no right or wrong way to grieve and there is no timeline on the grief you may experience. It is important that if you are sad, that you give yourself the time and space needed to grieve or spend time in mourning. This process cannot be sped up or skipped. You must allow yourself time to grieve in order to move forward.

You may be surprised with how you feel especially if you felt that miscarriage was not a big deal prior to your own personal loss. You may show very little grief in the early days but experience intense grief months or even years later. This is normal. This just means everyone grieves differently. Some may never grieve the loss of their baby. This is okay too. It is important not to feel bad if your feelings are not as intense as someone else's.

The father of the baby may react differently then what you would expect and this can cause friction between the two of you. Try to keep in mind that everyone grieves differently. Even if he isn't mourning the loss, he may still be upset, it just may not be in ways you can see.

Another common reaction is feeling like you are still pregnant. It takes time for the body to return to the pre-pregnant state and sometimes you may forget that you miscarried. You may find yourself still rubbing your belly, avoiding things that would have been harmful during pregnancy and possibly yearning to hold a baby. This is normal too, although it can be emotionally painful.

Some women purchase a teddy bear or other stuffed doll and carry it to help with the yearning to hold a baby. There are weighted bears specifically for this, such as Molly Bears or the bears available through HEALing Embrace.

You may be worried that you will never feel normal or like yourself again. You may wonder when the sadness will go away. There is no way to tell how long you will feel sad. This is discussed in more detail in the recovering chapter.

Emotional Expression

You may feel emotional, weepy, confused, tearful, anxious, easily upset, overly sensitive, irritable, angry, nervous, very tired, or a vast array of other emotions. All of these feelings are normal. It takes time to heal both emotionally and physically following the loss of a baby. Be gentle with yourself as you navigate through these feelings.

Grief can be very isolating. Mothers often find comfort in a place where they can openly express their grief and find acknowledgment for their pain. Cry with someone. Connect with someone who seems to understand. They may or may not have experienced a pregnancy loss but if they offer to be the shoulder for you, they can be very comforting.

At the end of this book, a few resources for support are listed but there are many more available. Your local hospital or hospice may have their own support group specific for miscarriage as well.

Physical Reactions

You can also have physical reactions to grief such as heart palpitations, insomnia, headaches, loss of appetite, inability to concentrate, withdrawal from friends and family or events and stomachaches. Some women have had a physical aching in their arms due to the desire to hold and nurture their baby.

Many women report having scary dreams or nightmares. This can occur both before the loss and after. Some women who had dreams of their baby dying prior to the miscarriage look back and believe this dream was preparing them.

Time Off for Miscarriage

It is important that you take time away from work for as long as you can and for as long as you feel you need. Talk with your employer and request as much time off as possible.

Depending on your employer, time off for a miscarriage may be covered under FMLA (Family Medical Leave Act); however, keep in mind that FMLA does not necessarily mean you will have paid time off. Some employers allow the use of sick time and/or vacation time to provide a paycheck during FMLA leave. Check with your HR department to determine your employer's policy.

In addition, the requested time off under FMLA would not be recognized as time off due to the birth of a child. The most common condition that has been accepted for time off due to miscarriage is defined by FMLA as a:

> Serious health condition" which means an illness, injury, impairment, or physical or mental condition that involves: "a period of incapacity requiring absence of more

than three calendar days from work, school, or other regular daily activities that also involves continuing treatment by (or under the supervision of) a health care provider.

You will need to work with a therapist or your obstetrician to complete the necessary paperwork to take this time off and be protected by FMLA. Your spouse may also qualify and file for FMLA. Have your spouse check with their HR department.

Even though you may be experiencing the emotional anguish that follows pregnancy loss, you must keep in mind that you have just given birth and your body will need time to recover. If you don't feel comfortable taking time off because of your emotional or mental state, it is perfectly acceptable to request time off due to the healing your body needs. You may be bleeding and cramping for several days or longer. If you had given birth at full-term, you would need at least two to four weeks to recover from birth. You may also lactate (make breast milk) even in an early miscarriage. Every woman's body is different and responds differently. You may go through the same emotional roller coaster that women experience following a full-term birth.

Remember, every pregnant woman, regardless of whether or not her baby is born alive or dead, needs time to heal. Your body has produced hormones and adjusted in ways we don't fully understand or know. Your body can't go back to a pre-pregnant state immediately.

Many work situations are not accommodating to regular crying spells, so it is recommended that you wait to go back until you're past the early weepy stages of the postpartum hormonal changes and grief. If you aren't feeling better in two to three weeks, seek professional help. Be kind to yourself. Know that grief is hard and it can take a long time to feel normal again.

Other Reasons to Take Time Off Work

You may need to take some time planning on how you might deal with any questions or hurtful comments from coworkers. It may be helpful for you to send out a mass email to your co-workers explaining what happened and give them ideas on what they can say to you to support you through this loss. Be sure you check your company policy to ensure you are not violating a policy. Some employers do not allow you to send out mass emails. You can also send this email to friends and family. It's perfectly acceptable for you to explain in the email exactly what they should and shouldn't say to you.

It's okay for you to educate people about how their comments can be more helpful. You can be very specific and let people know that they can say comments such as, "I am so sorry for your loss. I am here for you." Let them know you may just need to talk or cry and it's okay that they just listen and not try to fix things. You can also tell them in the email what not to say, such as, "You can always have another." "It was God's plan." "It's nature's way of dealing with a sick baby." "You already have a child and should feel blessed." Sometimes people say those things, trying to make you feel better, but in the end those comments usually do more harm than good. It's appropriate for you to let people know that.

Remember that these comments aren't meant to be hurtful. Situations like this make others uncomfortable. Miscarriage is very common, but many women are left to grieve in silence. You might be surprised to learn your friend or co-worker also had a loss.

Saying It

I lost a baby. My baby died. My daughter passed away. I have one living child. It's hard at first and can be awkward. Being able to acknowledge what happened and to say it aloud may make it more real and easier to accept.

If you're afraid to tell people what happened, try not to be. It can be very healing for you to say it out loud. If you don't feel like you need to say it, that's okay too. What's important is that you do what feels right for you.

If you named your baby, it can be very healing to call your baby by their given name. Encourage others to do so.

Chapter Five: Causes

Did I Cause This?

Women often search for a reason for the miscarriage. A reason for miscarriage is found less than 50% of the time. Many women will blame themselves and feel they did something to cause the miscarriage. Previous abortion(s) or prior use of birth control has not been shown to cause miscarriage. Physical exercise/exertion, sports, or working does not cause miscarriage. Below is a list of things known not to cause miscarriage:

- Anxiety
- Sexual intercourse
- Travel
- Lifting
- Occasional use of alcohol or over-the-counter medications
- Exhaust fumes

Why Did This Happen?

Oftentimes, parents want to know why their baby died or why the miscarriage happened. Only about 50% of the time is a cause found. Some families find comfort in not knowing and others struggle when they don't have a reason. Most miscarriages are not caused by anything you did.

Below are some listed causes of miscarriage.

- Failure of the egg to properly implant into the lining of the uterus.
- The number one cited reason for miscarriage before 12 weeks gestation is a genetic abnormality with the baby. While the cells were dividing, sometimes DNA translocates or causes a genetic error which results in the baby developing incorrectly. There is no known way to prevent a genetic error.
- Low progesterone is another common reason for miscarriage. This can be diagnosed during the pregnancy. While some studies do not show that supplementation with progesterone prevents miscarriage, there is low risk to taking progesterone supplementation. Progesterone is an important hormone which supports a pregnancy. Progesterone thickens the lining of the uterus which is where the very early and developing baby implants and receives its nutrients in order to grow. With low levels of progesterone, a baby may not have the nutrients needed to support it until the placenta grows and takes over this important function.
- Uterine anomalies are another cause of miscarriage. An anomaly could be scar tissue in the uterus from a

previous abortion or D&C procedure, endometriosis, uterine infection, C-section or other uterine surgery, fibroids, polyps or other uterine growths, septate uterus, or how your uterus developed in your mother's womb.

- Incompetent cervix is another cause of miscarriage. This is where the cervix, which is the opening of your uterus, cannot hold the weight of the baby and dilates (opens) and effaces (softens, shortens and becomes thinner) early. The baby would then be born (alive or deceased) but would be too premature for healthcare providers to utilize any life-saving measures. An incompetent cervix is most often diagnosed in the second trimester although some women have experienced an incompetent cervix earlier. Sometimes in a threatened miscarriage, this issue can be diagnosed and treated, but most often, it is not treated until a subsequent pregnancy. Treatment includes surgically closing the cervix with a purse-string type stitch known as a cervical cerclage. These stitches are removed once you reach full term.

- Blood disorders are also a reason for miscarriage. Blood disorders that affect clotting are common but women are often not tested for these clotting and antigen disorders until they have had several early miscarriages. Some of these disorders can be treated with medications in subsequent pregnancies.

- Very rarely, infections can cause miscarriage. Infections such as Rubella or untreated bacterial infections have caused miscarriage.

Will This Happen Again?

If a treatable condition is found and treated in future pregnancies, the risk of miscarriage decreases, however, there is always a risk. Your chances of having a successful pregnancy following a miscarriage are about the same as if you had never had a miscarriage in the past. You may need additional monitoring in future pregnancies, but many women go on to have healthy babies.

Chapter Six: Others Who Grieve

Your Grieving Partner

While women experience an emotional and physical loss, men will only experience the emotional loss. They won't experience the cramps, feeling that their bodies failed, leaky breasts, or the return of menstruation; but your partner will most likely experience some level of emotional grief. Some of the feelings men have are anger, denial, feelings of helplessness, loss of control, disbelief, uselessness and guilt. Many men also feel like their partner will die. This is common with any birth complication and it is no different with pregnancy loss.

Your partner will watch you go through an experience he may not fully understand and it may make him uncomfortable to realize he cannot take away any of the emotional or physical pain. He may not ask questions because he does not understand medical terms or is uncomfortable. He may suppress his grief in order to support you.

You may also get frustrated with him because he may not seem to grieve. It's very common for men to grieve differently than women or for people who didn't experience the loss on a physical level to grieve differently. Men tend to grieve in a more private way. It can also be very difficult for you if your partner wasn't attached to the pregnancy. For an early loss, the only attachment your partner may have is an ultrasound picture. He didn't experience food cravings, nausea, or a growing belly with kicks and punches. You may feel at times like you're grieving alone.

Women have reported that their partners seemed to retreat. Many became involved in projects such as building things or fixing up the house. Some partners completely sink into their work or withdraw — going in early and staying late. They might work long hours, pick up extra shifts and seem like they are avoiding the home.

Some men will outwardly mourn their loss. You may see them cry, which can be painful for you. It is also very common for men to seem stoic in the first few months following the loss but to regress three to six months later. This is due to pent up emotions and your partner finally being able to release his grief. Society also pushes the attitude that men shouldn't cry because it shows weakness. We know that not to be true but sometimes men suppress their feelings to fall in line with this societal attitude. In addition, men sometimes feel left out since much of the attention is placed on the woman's grief.

It is important to check in with him. Ask him questions and let him know you need support and that you are there to support him as well. Make sure you tell him specific ways he can support you. Tell him you need him to hold you, talk with you, or ask you questions about what you're experiencing. He needs to know how to help you. He may have never been through this before and he cannot read your mind. He'll need guidance on how to help you. Also ask him how you can help him in his grief. Maybe he needs another man to talk with and you can help by asking your support groups and other people about support groups for men? Maybe he needs space each day to be on his own? Be sure to find out what his needs are too.

Some men resort to smoking, alcohol and drugs. This is an unhealthy way to grieve and it is important that you both seek counseling and assistance. It can be difficult for men to talk out these feelings, but there are many men only groups as well as men who have been through miscarriage and stillbirth who are open to talking with other men about their experiences. Online support groups are very popular for men and there are many men specific blogs out there as well.

Your Living Children

Children grieve too. If you told your children about your pregnancy and experienced the loss with them, there are books for children on miscarriage which can be helpful. Some children may feel guilty as if they caused the loss somehow. Guilt can appear regardless of whether or not the child didn't want a brother or sister or a child that said they only wanted a sister and the baby was a brother and vice versa.

Grief can manifest in stomachaches, headaches and disagreements in school or with friends. Grief in children comes in many forms. It can be helpful to find group therapy or a therapist that specializes in child grief.

If you didn't share your pregnancy with your children, they'll sense that something is wrong no matter how hard you try to hide your feelings and emotions. When children see their parents try to hide their pain, it can be very scary for them. Your child(ren) most likely have never seen you or your partner this way before. It is very important to talk with them and share with them in terms they can understand. You know your child(ren) best; reveal to them what you feel is age appropriate.

If you can't find the words, purchase a book. Most are storylines that are age appropriate. They can be difficult to read because of your emotional state, but they can help put the words in your mouth that you have struggled to find.

If you're having intense feelings of guilt, try to take some time out for your children . . . but understand you're not superwoman and this will be a small blip on their screen years later. Do your best to help them understand what you're experiencing and talk with them about their experience. Remember that this is not your fault. You did not cause this grief your child is experiencing. You do not need to move on quickly in order to make life return to normal for you and your family. Children will see that it is okay to grieve and mourn by watching the way you grieve and mourn. Your life will most likely never feel the same, but happiness will return. Children will see this as well, which will help them feel safe with their feelings.

Future Children

If or when you choose to have another baby, they will not replace the baby that died. You will have to decide if you want to share your pregnancy loss with your future children. The when and how you will do it may vary. Some families share from the beginning. They always talk about their deceased baby; they may have pictures in their home, mementos, or other important items they share. There are also books available that can help put this experience into words. Books can be a healing way to introduce the deceased sibling to future siblings.

Chapter Seven: Sharing the News

Sharing Your Loss with Others (How to Tell Your Family and Friends)

You may feel compelled to announce your miscarriage or baby's death. You most likely have announced your pregnancy, so announcing your baby's death seems proper. The big question is how?

A standard baby announcement won't work. Some people have adapted their announcement from a standard baby announcement. You could choose a picture such as an ultrasound photo or even a picture of a pregnancy test. Then find a statement. Obituaries and memorial quotes can be helpful. If you named your baby, you may place your baby's name on the announcement followed by you and your partner's name and the name of any siblings. The death date can be placed on the announcement or you can use the conception date (if known) to the death date. The death date and birth date may be different. You can put both dates on the announcement or pick the one for you that has the most meaning.

Many women find it appropriate to send the announcement to close friends and family members. There are many different ways to announce and honor your baby. If you feel compelled to make an announcement, take your time putting it together. You can have these printed at any of your local print stores or they can be printed online. Sending an email announcement, placing an obituary in the newspaper, or announcing over social media are also methods families have used.

At elizabethpetrucelli.com, you will find a post titled "Announcing a Miscarriage on Facebook," that is extremely helpful.

How Others May React

Friends and Family

You won't be able to lean on every friend, sister, mother, or family member. This event won't affect them the same way it's affected you. You will learn quickly who you can lean on for support and who you want to avoid. You may even be surprised by some of the people who will be there for you and find disappointment in the people you thought would be there but seemed to disappear. It is not uncommon to lose friendships during and after pregnancy loss. It's okay to let them go. Focus on the friends who are there for you. You need support and you can't be worried about a friend being upset with you because you're grieving. Your grief won't look like anyone else's. There is no right way to grieve. Just allow yourself to do it.

It may seem like the best person to lean on is someone who has experienced pregnancy loss; however, use caution. Not all pregnancy loss mothers feel pain in their loss and some may not want to share their pain with you. Mothers who are willing to share their pain and allow you into their lives will make themselves known to you.

Family and friends may feel very uncomfortable. The death of a child isn't supposed to happen. It is not the natural order of life. Due to this internal discomfort, people often say the "wrong" things believing they are helpful. Because of this, try not to take their silence or inappropriate comments personally. Be prepared to be assertive and set boundaries. It's okay to express what you need and what you don't need. If someone makes an inappropriate comment, it's okay to tell them. Most people aren't trying to be malicious or hurtful; they just don't know what to do.

In the back of this book, you can tear out the pages with the following information. They can be easily handed to friends and family or placed on a countertop or other public area for all to see.

Help Them Help You

What to Say

"I don't know what to say."

"Who can I call for you?" (Be prepared to actually make those phone calls).

"Be patient with yourself. Grief has no timeline."

"Don't feel guilty because you laughed today."

"Can I take your baby's siblings to the park? I know you don't feel like laughing or playing right now."

"I am going to the store, can I bring anything back for you?"

"Talk to me. I am here to listen."

"I am out running errands, is there anything you need?"

"How are you doing today?"

"You don't have to answer the phone or call me back, I just wanted to check in on you."

"How about I take your baby's siblings to school, or grandma's, or ____?"

"I would love to attend a support group with you or go to church with you."

What Not to Say

"You can have another baby."

"At least you know you can get pregnant."

"It was God's way of protecting you from ____."

"It was God's will."

"Heaven needed another angel."

"Your baby is better in Heaven."

"Time heals all wounds."

"I know just how you feel." (Unless you have personally experienced pregnancy loss).

"It could have been worse."

"Now you have an angel/saint in Heaven."

"You should be over this by now! It's been _____
weeks/months/years."
"God never gives us more than we can handle."
"What can I do for you?" Instead say, "Can I do ___ for
you? Or "I am going to bring over a meal" not "Can I bring
over a meal?"

Ways They Can Help

- Listen –You may want to talk over and over again
  about the pregnancy and the death experience. Finding
  someone who will listen no matter how many times you
  need to share is important. . Most people want to stop
  listening after the 3rd or 4th time.
- Bring tissues.
- Give you a hug.
- Encourage you to have pictures taken with your baby.
- Ask and hold your baby.
- Be a shoulder to cry on. If you don't want to talk, you
  may just want someone to lean on while you cry.
- Cry with you. They don't have to be stoic. Crying helps
  validate that this is a sad time and an experience worth
  grieving.
- Be there – For the birth that is. If they would have most
  likely been there for the birth anyway, be sure to let
  them know you would still like them to be there to
  support you. At the very least, you may prefer they wait
  in the waiting room
- Call your baby by name – which may seem weird at
  first. This is the preferred method unless you do not
  want them to call your baby by name.

- Mementos – Bring something for you to remember your baby by. For any birth, people give gifts. This is no different although the gifts might be slightly different. You may want an outfit.. Families are often encouraged to dress their baby just like they would if the baby was born alive. A teddy bear that is at least 14 inches but less than 24 inches is best as well. You can hold the bear as you leave the hospital. If you provide the baby's weight, they can make a bear of the same weight. Anything with the baby's name or birthstone on it, such as jewelry, is also customary. Cards are also welcome and can be kept as a keepsake. Any of the traditional keepsakes will also work such as something to preserve a lock of hair, handprints/footprints, molds and books or special boxes to keep pictures in.
- Have them make phone calls for you.
- They can send a card. There is a line of cards for pregnancy and infant loss by Hallmark and other card makers.
- Be comfortable in your tears.
- Attend the funeral/memorial service.
- Send a daily message but they should not expect a response. "How are you today?" "Thinking of you." "Hope things are going okay."
- Understand that the next year will be a "year of firsts." Going into your home without your baby will be a "first," returning to work will be a "first," going to the same grocery store will be a "first," and any holiday will be a "first" holiday without your baby. There will be many "firsts."
- Remember the baby's birthday/angel date/death date. Send a card, make a phone call, send a text. It can be as

simple as "Remembering your baby's (can insert baby's name) birth today."

- Remember the baby's due date – If your baby died before their due date, this will be a particularly difficult day. They can let your know they are thinking of you and that they are there for you.
- Be supportive in the weeks and months to come.
- Attend memorial events – Be there for the funeral or any memorial events and find local walks and other annual remembrance events to help share and remember your baby.
- Set up a meal train/calendar of people who will bring you meals. Soups can be hearty and healthy. Bringing veggie trays, fruit trays, sandwich trays, or just setting out some healthy food can be extremely helpful. It is a reminder that you need to eat, which is often put on hold while mourning.
- Bring household items such as milk, eggs, butter, toilet paper, paper towels, paper plates, aluminum foil, toothpaste, etc.
- Mow the lawn, take out the trash, bring in the trash cans, etc.
- Pick up around the house (do laundry, mow the lawn, empty and load the dishwasher, make the beds, etc). They should not break down the baby's nursery or remove any items for the baby.

Chapter Eight:
Remembering Your Baby

Remembering Your Baby

Funeral or Memorial Service

Regardless of what you choose to do with the physical form of your baby's body, you can still hold a funeral or memorial service. If you aren't getting any options for local burial and cremation, call a local funeral home or your church. Some cemeteries have communal plots. You may also contact the Catholic diocese in your area to see if they have a location. You don't have to be Catholic to ask about their communal burial options.

A memorial can be appropriate and very healing. If this is something you desire, you can either send out invitations or call your friends and family members and ask them to come to the service. The service might look similar to a wake. There could be flowers and a table displaying your baby's name, pictures of your pregnancy, ultrasound pictures and other items you may have to remember your baby. A sign-in book can also be bought and you could add this to your memory box. Prayers or thoughts/poems could be read to those who attend and there could be an opportunity for people to come forward and talk. A memorial service doesn't have to look like anything specific, so trust what feels right to you.

If you flushed any tissue, fetal remains, or your baby, a water ceremony may help you if you are struggling with this. At the website elizabethpetrucelli.com, you will find instructions on the water ceremony for miscarriage.

Should I Name My Baby?

Some women feel called to name their baby but this doesn't mean you have to. If you feel it's important to you, go ahead and find an appropriate name. If your partner doesn't feel this is necessary, discuss why you feel it's important and ask if they would be okay if you chose a name. It doesn't matter how far along you were when you experienced your loss. You had hopes and dreams and aspirations for this baby. Some of you may have already been picking out names.

Some of you may have been so early in your pregnancy that it would be impossible to know the sex. If you feel compelled to name your baby, you can either choose a name that's not gender specific or you can choose a name based on the sex of the baby your intuition has prompted you toward. Some people choose a first name and middle name of the opposite sex such as Mary Joseph or Matthew Elizabeth.

Rituals

For many, it can be healing to do something to honor your experience and your baby on your baby's expected due date or other dates that seem significant. There are many options. Some people plant a tree. Some release balloons, light a candle, pick flowers and send them down a stream. Some will take the day off and spend it in nature.

Some people also get a memorial plaque made, a birthstone, or donate to a charitable organization. There are also organizations that put together bereavement walks for pregnancy loss. They focus on bereavement care, resources and support for those touched by different types of loss, including miscarriage, stillbirth, or neonatal death.

There are annual candlelight vigils on October 15th all over the world in honor of Pregnancy and Infant Loss Remembrance Day. Since the holidays can be a difficult time for many, some families pick a charity to donate to in honor of their baby or they participate in an Angel Tree or Adopt a Family/Child and shop for a child that would be the same age as their baby. This can be very comforting and healing.

Baby Book

With a miscarriage, their might not be many tangible items of your baby or anything your baby touched, but many families create a book and put the following items inside: positive pregnancy test, lab results, ultrasound photos, hospital band from D&C, completed journal, pictures drawn, poems, work from therapy, the birth announcement, pictures their siblings made and the sympathy cards received.

A baby book or a memory box is a great way to keep all your important mementos together. Some families are able to include: pictures from labor and birth, along with a lock of hair. Other suitable items might be pictures or cards from your baby shower, the outfit you were planning on bringing your baby home in, your baby's band, your hospital band and handprints and/or footprints. Other items from the hospital, such as a baby blanket, can also be placed in the book or box. Some hospitals dress babies who pass. You can place your baby's clothes in the book or box.

Whatever you choose, it's important that it feels right to you. If you're reading this as you're experiencing your loss, keep in mind you might not be in an emotional state to make these decisions, and that's okay. If you didn't get any of these mementos or you weren't given options, this may be difficult for you.

You won't go back in the baby book for positive memories, you'll be visiting the book to remember your child. There is no right or wrong way. Everyone will use their baby book differently.

Mother's Day

It's hard for most women to believe they're a mother if they have no living children. You conceived a child in your womb and did all the right things for that child. Many of you prayed for that child's health, and many of you may feel guilty thinking that you did something that may have caused this. Your baby didn't die because of anything you did. It still doesn't change the fact that you had a child, and that child died. Celebrate Mother's Day in whatever way feels right for you.

Other Ways to Remember and Memorialize Your Baby

Some grieving mothers and grieving fathers get a tattoo. It could be your baby's name, a butterfly or other creature that represents your baby, or a replica of your baby's hand/footprints. If this doesn't sound like something you'd like to do, you could also buy a bracelet, necklace, or ring.

Chapter Nine:
Recovering

Recovering

Postpartum

You were pregnant. Now you're not. It doesn't matter if you had a living baby or your baby passed, your body will be in a postpartum state. There are hormone changes that take place in a woman's body that can affect her emotions.

The same warnings for postpartum depression apply after a pregnancy loss. In fact, 12% of women will experience depression and 20% will experience a combination of depression and grief (you can study the reference material for this data at the end of the book). Grief is normal and you may experience all the stages of grief — denial, anger, guilt, depression and acceptance.

If you're feeling sad and weepy for longer than two weeks, are feeling no desire to live, have had thoughts of suicide, or have planned your suicide, seek treatment immediately.

If you experience the last two symptoms, you need to check into an emergency department immediately. Grief may last a long time, but you shouldn't be weepy every hour of every day. The weepiness should gradually improve. Even if you spent five minutes less weeping today versus yesterday, that's improvement. You will feel better. If you don't feel your enthusiasm for life returning, you should seek help from a professional.

You may bleed or spot for few weeks, you may experience cramping, your period may not resume for several weeks, and you may produce milk or experience breast engorgement (see reference materials). You also have pregnancy hormones in your body that could take months to get out of your system.

Due to your body changing from a pregnant state to a non-pregnant state, you may not want to have sex for a long time. Talk with your partner about this. It's just like after you have a baby. Your vagina may hurt, you may be bleeding and you may feel this could lead you down the road to another failed pregnancy. Your hormones will be off kilter because they are going back to a pre-pregnancy state. This is all normal. If it's debilitating for you, contact your doctor or OB/GYN. It shouldn't be years before you feel like having sex again, but a few months isn't atypical.

Lactation

Your body is prepared to breastfeed your baby by the fifth month; however, some women report producing milk with a loss as early as 12 weeks. Your body doesn't know your baby has died and may produce milk, even if you have never breastfed a baby before. This can be both physically and emotionally painful, or it can be very healing. If lactation occurs, you will typically feel engorgement sometime between days two and five, following your loss. Engorgement is a painful swelling of your breasts due to milk production. Many women describe this feeling as "breasts like rocks."

You have two options:

- Drying up
- Donating

Drying Up

It doesn't matter what option you choose but try not to feel guilty if you choose to dry up. Many women will bind their breasts and take ibuprofen to relieve some of the pain; however, binding is no longer recommended and may carry risk of developing clogged ducts and mastitis. It is recommended that you wear a bra and use cold packs and raw cabbage leaves. Place the raw or frozen cabbage leaves in your bra like breast pads. Wear them until they wilt. You can replace these several times a day. Please note that it is important not to use heat on your breasts during the time of engorgement as it can increase pain and swelling.

You will also want to avoid any nipple stimulation such as letting the shower water spray onto your breasts. There are herbs that can help dry milk and other natural remedies. Please consult an herbalist and discuss these options with your care provider.

You may need to pump or hand express a little milk in order to relieve some of the pressure. If this is the case, use an electric pump, manual pump, or hand express for two to three minutes. Pumping or expressing for much longer may stimulate milk production and delay the drying up process. Any milk collected can be stored in the freezer, poured down the drain, or donated to a milk bank (if you qualify). You may also send your milk to a company to have it preserved and turned into jewelry.

While you are waiting for your milk to dry up (which can take several days to weeks), breast pads can help absorb any leaking. Most stores carry disposable breast pads but there are also reusable cloth pads that can be purchased online or at breastfeeding specialty stores. If the thought of going to the store to purchase these items is painful, ask someone else to pick them up for you.

Donating

While some women prefer to donate, it is a commitment and involves applying and being accepted by a milk bank. At the time of this publication, there are 18 human milk banks in the United States and Canada. Visit https://www.hmbana.org/ to locate a milk bank near your area. You do not have to be near a milk bank to donate. Many will accept your donation from other states. You will need to apply and qualify as a donor. There are several steps in this process. They are:

- Call or email an inquiry to the milk bank.
- Participate in an eligibility interview.

- Complete a lifestyle history and medical review.
- Complete a medical release form which will need to be signed by your doctor.
- Consent to and receive blood tests for HIV, HTLV, Syphilis, Hepatitis C and Hepatitis B.

There is also a specific way that milk will need to be collected and sterilization of parts that will need to be adhered to. In addition, you will need to agree to the human milk bank guidelines in their information packet which describes acceptable use of over-the-counter medications, drugs, alcohol, smoking, caffeine, herbs and vitamins.

If you do not qualify for milk bank donation, you can privately donate your milk. There are several private donation websites and groups available on the internet. You do not have to pump for any length of time.

If you are choosing to donate, you will need an electric breast pump. A manual breast pump may be used as can manual expression but not if you are donating to a human milk bank. You can ask the hospital if you can borrow or rent one, but there are private businesses that will rent pumps if the hospital doesn't have one available. You can also purchase a pump at any store that sells them.

If you just want to pump to relieve engorgement and pressure, you can store just that amount of milk and donate it, or you can continue to pump and donate regularly. (See tear-out on breast milk storage). You can also create a keepsake with your milk through an organization that preserves milk. It is a wonderful memento that can remind you of your baby and the pregnancy.

Some women find comfort in donating when they know their milk will go to a baby in need. Donating milk to a human milk bank provides milk to sick and premature babies. This can be a living gift to another baby and their parents.

If you want to pump for any length of time, you will need storage containers and/or breast milk bags. Pump every three to four hours. The milk collected can be added to any milk already stored in a refrigerator but do not pour warm milk into a container with frozen milk. You will receive instructions on how to pump and store milk from the milk bank if you are qualified to donate.

Some women have found it comforting to pump every few hours and throughout the night because they are doing something that any mother would do if she had just had a baby. Others do not want to wake up and pump so they only pump during the day. If your goal is to pump long term, you will still need to pump during the night to maintain a milk supply.

It is important to really listen to your own desires. You do not have to do any of this if you do not want to. Even if you agree to donate milk and then decide it is too hard or too much, you can stop at any time. If you choose to stop though, you will need to slowly wean by increasing the time in between pumps and decreasing the time you pump. If you stop cold turkey you may become engorged and experience pain or develop clogged ducts and/or mastitis (breast infection).

If you had been pumping every three hours for about 20 minutes, try pumping every four to five hours and only for

15 minutes. Continue to decrease the length of the pumping and increase the time in between pumps over several days. You will dry up within a few days to a few weeks. The goal is to gradually decrease pumping and not just stop altogether.

If you have questions or concerns about drying up your milk or donating, contact your doctor or hospital's lactation consultant or find a local lactation consultant to assist you.

Warning Signs:

Sore, painful, reddened area in your breast or armpit area (sign of mastitis/breast infection). Contact your care provider if you experience any of these symptoms.

Baby Samples, Magazines and More

If you signed up for baby samples, pregnancy magazines, or other free items, you will receive items for months and possibly years following your loss. Some women don't have to sign up online because their doctor's office will sign them up at the first prenatal visit.

Unfortunately, many of these companies share your information, so the news spreads and you soon find yourself with stacks of samples and magazines in addition to an email box full of mail telling you all about the development of your baby next week. These can be hurtful reminders of what you lost.

If you remember where you signed up, you can return to the website and unsubscribe, but if you don't, it may be best to enlist your partner, friend, or family member to assist you in calling the companies or fishing through your emails to unsubscribe to all these reminders. At the bottom of the email, you will find an area that says something similar to "to unsubscribe, click here." By clicking that link, you will either be unsubscribed or be directed to enter the email address that you would like unsubscribed. You can also visit http://www.privacyrights.org/fs/fs4-junk.htm#MPS

Or send a letter plus a $1 check or money order to:

> Mail Preference Service
> Direct Marketing Association
> PO Box 643
> Carmel, NY 10512

Another aspect to remember will be the hospital bills that come in several weeks and even months after the loss. If your husband or partner can pay those up front for you, this may help alleviate reliving those memories. You can also contact your insurance companies or the doctors and ask them to send the bills addressed to your husband only.

Recovery

Grief is painful, but it is possible to move forward . . . when one is ready. Some women feel they have moved through their grief after only a week and other women are still grieving decades after their loss. Again, grief has no timeline.

At some point, you will most likely feel some sense of normalcy again. Some women describe feeling guilty when they start to feel normal or like themselves again, as if that means they have somehow betrayed their lost one. When you begin to feel more at peace with your loss, remember it is okay to feel this and that you are not betraying your baby. Remember that moving forward and rejoining the living doesn't mean that you have forgotten your loss and its impact. You will have good days and bad days, and then one day you might come to realize that you are having more good days than bad. Only then will you know you are normal again.

Journaling

Journaling can help in so many ways. You can journal each day, several times a day, or only once a week. It doesn't matter how often you journal. When you have to deal with something difficult, your journal can be a companion to you. There is no right or wrong way to journal. You can journal about the happy moments as well as the sad ones. You can journal about what your baby may look like. You can even draw your baby and make that part of your journal. Your journal can be filled with letters to your baby or you can talk about the medical aspects of your loss and any other struggles you're having.

Your journal can hold whatever needs to be released. Journaling also helps to take some of the pressure off your partner. While your partner most likely wants to help you, he may not want to hear the story over and over again. Many women type their journal in a blog or word processing program, but if you prefer, you can write in a nice journal book or any old notebook. Go with what feels good to you.

Therapy

It can be very helpful to find a good therapist or support group. Many support groups are free. Attending a support group can help you validate your own grief and know that it is okay to be in pain. Some groups are large, others are small, but it is important that you find a group that fits your needs. Some women do not want to attend a group where women are sharing their loss story at every session. If this concerns you, check with the group leader to see how they manage story sharing and if there are healing activities and other discussion when processing loss.

If you are concerned about your emotional state and feel "crazy," or have been told you need to seek professional help, there are many therapists you can see that specialize in grief. It is also important to find a therapist you like and who meshes with you. They do not necessarily have to specialize in miscarriage or perinatal loss, although some therapists specialize in this area. You may be able to find recommendations from support group members, other friends and family, or by calling local support organizations in your area.

Chapter Ten: Re-entering Society

Relief often follows the experience of miscarriage. If you felt an impending miscarriage and it's not over, relief is a common feeling. This can be confusing, especially when grief returns following the relief. It is okay to feel relieved. You have survived the miscarriage and life will go on.

After experiencing miscarriage, when it's time to go to the store, go back to work, or just go out, there will be reminders of the pregnancy everywhere. Even the grocery store clerk might have known you were pregnant. You may have had a growing belly and now your belly is flat or flabby. Being prepared for how to handle these encounters is important.

When a person asks and discovers you are no longer pregnant, they may also feel devastated for you. It is not your responsibility to make them feel better or comfort them. Many women do, but know that you cannot control their feelings and try not to feel guilty for sharing your story.

Going Back to Work

Telling your co-workers, clients, students, or others that you interact with at work can be challenging. One of the most common ways to share your news is via email or letter. You can send a scripted letter/email to your co-workers or have your supervisor send out the message. The message should be short but explain the situation and include how you are feeling now. By including how you are feeling, it will help your co-workers understand where you are in your journey and how to help you at that stage. You could even include the list of what to say and not to say in your message.

Going back at the end of the workweek instead of the beginning has also shown to be very helpful. This gives you that "light at the end of the tunnel" feeling where you know that you only have a day or so until the weekend where you can recover. Scheduling self-care for that first weekend is also important. A massage, mani/pedi, date night, night out with friends, or a night in with a warm blanket and a special movie can help you feel better after a stressful week at work.

Refer to the tear-out at the back of this book that can help you tell others about your loss.

Going Out in Public

It is inevitable. You will have to go out in public at some point. There are people who may have known that you were pregnant and will either ask you how the baby is or how the pregnancy is going or notice that your belly has gotten smaller. Having a canned response can be very helpful during these encounters. Many women felt more comfortable with those first few outings when they have a friend or someone with them to help deflect the comments or step in should emotions take over.

As you navigate the public again, you will one day be asked how many children you have or if you plan on having any children. Some women share their story of loss with others easily yet others struggle to share. Sometimes random strangers have a difficult time understanding and the roles change where the grieving parent feels they need to comfort and reassure the stranger. Finding balance in who you share with and what you share will be helpful. It's okay not to tell every person you come in contact with, just as much as it's perfectly fine to tell every person you come in contact with. Some women like to practice what they will say ahead of time and have found that it made encounters less awkward. It is also important to be kind to yourself if you don't share your experience with your child and begin to feel guilty. You may not always share your child and that's okay. If you find you are feeling guilty about this, writing a letter to your child can help, or share your story the next time you are out.

Others Who Are Pregnant

You will cross paths with other women who are pregnant, even within your close family. This can be difficult as you navigate your new normal. You might be expected to put on a baby shower or at the very least, attend a baby shower. If it doesn't feel right, it is important to not do it. Don't push yourself to be there for someone else. Talk with this pregnant mother and share your feelings. She may not understand, but your emotional health is more important.

Trust your gut and stay home if that's what feels right. You may also notice that your pregnant friends stop sharing their pregnancy news with you. Many do this because they don't want to hurt you. They are unsure what to do or say to you. If it bothers you, share those feelings as well.

Many loss mothers temporarily remove themselves from social media sites so they can get a reprieve from all the baby announcements, pregnancy complaints and pictures of new baby's. It's okay to remove yourself for a period of time. When it feels right, you can pick up where you left off. It is okay to stay away from pregnant friends or friends with children because it is too painful.

Chapter Eleven:
Pregnancy After Loss

Pregnancy Following a Loss

Fear of enduring another miscarriage is one of the biggest concerns women have during their pregnancy after a loss. While you may feel more prepared than ever if you experienced another loss, you may still be hurting deeply from your previous loss and fear the pain you may experience again.

There are many factors that must be taken into consideration when deciding the right time to try again. Ensure you're talking with your care provider about the best time to try to conceive. Most care providers recommend that you experience a few cycles before attempting another pregnancy. While you may be physically ready to conceive, you must also be emotionally prepared for the journey.

Many women will go on to have another baby; however, some will not. Having another baby won't take away the sadness or grief you experience because of your loss. Some women may actually feel more guilt because they conceived again. This guilt may stem from feeling like you haven't grieved the loss completely and are attempting to replace the baby, or because you conceived too soon. These are all normal feelings.

You can write a letter to your new baby or a letter to the baby you lost and explain your feelings. This can be very therapeutic. Putting your thoughts on paper and re-reading them really helps make sense of them.

You may also have doubts about your care provider or insurance company. It will be important for you to find a care provider you can trust. If you have the option of care provider shopping, find a care provider you trust and reveal your prior loss(es) to them. This will build not only trust in their abilities but will build trust in yourself that you can find a care provider for you and your baby.

You may also worry about this pregnancy. Many women experience anxiety during their subsequent pregnancies and then become concerned that this worry could be passed onto the new baby being carried. Try to focus on all the positive things that are taking place and acknowledge the wonder and awe of this current pregnancy. You may find it helpful to share the news of your pregnancy with trusted friends and family members so you have people you can count on for support when you're overly anxious.

Focus on lowering your stress level. Exercise can be extremely beneficial. Pregnancy yoga helps with breathing and builds strength. Many people can do pregnancy yoga over most other exercise. In addition, eat right and take time for yourself. Now could be the time to start regular pregnancy massages, acupuncture, chiropractic visits, or meditation. Many women use Hypnobirthing to help them focus on the positive aspects of their pregnancy. Another idea to help with bonding and reduce stress is to take a bath each day.

It is a rare person that takes time each day to focus on themselves but this is so important to help reduce your anxiety. Your partner can help by setting up the bathtub. Dim the lights, light some candles, turn on some soft music and relax in the warmth of the water. Rub your belly and talk to your baby. Really listen to your body and send positive messages to your baby. This will help counteract all the anxiety and negativity you have been feeling. For this moment, you are loving on your baby.

Bonding with your baby may be difficult. Despite the uncertainty, it's best to try to bond with the new baby. It will be hard, but you must try. If you fear bonding because of guilt, understand that nothing will replace the baby you lost. Each baby is an individual.

Visit PregnancyAfterLossSupport.com for amazing resources and support.

Chapter Twelve: Helping Someone Through Pregnancy Loss — Do's and Don'ts

Don't be silent. Silence can be extremely painful. They will remember your silence. There is a difference between active silence and silence that is to ignore. Ignoring silence means avoidance, rejection, minimization, rushing through the event, fear and silence because "this is so uncomfortable." Families feel supported in silence when there is active listening, attentiveness and presence (a shoulder to lean on). Don't just fill silence with jabber. It's okay to just sit with the family in silence, but do not ignore their pain.

Grief has no timeline. They will never forget. Don't put time limits on how long you think they should grieve. Don't disappear because you think you will "make them cry," or "make them remember." They want to remember and they will cry anyway. They will find comfort in you remembering.

The grief felt from losing a baby is not smaller because the baby is smaller. The empty place felt from a baby's death is never going to be filled. It's a pain that will never completely heal or be relieved by subsequent pregnancies. - Melinda Olsen, Earth Mama Angel Baby

The list below gives you many ideas on what to say and how to help. Keep in mind there is no one right thing to say or do.

What to Say

"I don't know what to say."

"Who can I call for you?" (Be prepared to actually make those phone calls).

"Be patient with yourself. Grief has no timeline."

"Don't feel guilty because you laughed today."

"Can I take your baby's siblings to the park? I know you don't feel like laughing or playing right now."

"I am going to the store, can I bring anything back for you?"

"Talk to me. I am here to listen."

"I am out running errands, is there anything you need?"

"How are you doing today?"

"You don't have to answer the phone or call me back, I just wanted to check in on you."

"How about I take your baby's siblings to school, or grandma's, or ____?"

"I would love to attend a support group with you or go to church with you."

What Not to Say

"You can have another baby."

"At least you know you can get pregnant."

"It was God's way of protecting you from ____."

"It was God's will."

"Heaven needed another angel."

"Your baby is better in Heaven."

"Time heals all wounds."

"I know just how you feel." (Unless you have personally experienced pregnancy loss).

"It could have been worse."

"Now you have an angel/saint in Heaven."

"You should be over this by now! It's been ____ weeks/months/years."

"God never gives us more than we can handle."

"What can I do for you?" Instead say, "Can I do ___ for you? Or "I am going to bring over a meal" not "Can I bring over a meal?"

Things You Can Do

- Listen – They may want to talk over and over again about the pregnancy and the death experience. Be the person they can go to and vent with and repeat their story. Most people want to stop listening after the 3rd or 4th time.
- Bring tissues.
- Give them a hug.
- Encourage the family to have pictures taken with their baby.
- Ask and hold the baby.

- Be their shoulder to cry on. If they don't want to talk, they may just want someone to lean on while they cry. Let them cry. Crying is just one way to express grief.
- Cry with them. You don't have to be stoic. Crying helps validate that this is a sad time and an experience worth grieving. They will not be angry with you for crying.
- Be there – For the birth that is. If you would have most likely been there for the birth anyway, be sure to let them know you would still like to be there to support them. At the very least, the family may prefer you wait in the waiting room (which can be typical at a live birth too).
- Call their baby by name – which may seem weird. Unless the family does not want you to call their baby by name, this is preferred.
- Mementos – Bring something for them to remember their baby by. For any birth, people give gifts. This is no different although the gifts might be slightly different. The family may want an outfit, so ask. Families are often encouraged to dress their baby just like they would at a live birth. A teddy bear that is at least 14 inches but less than 24 inches is best as well. Mom can hold the bear as she leaves the hospital. You can also find out the baby's weight and make a bear of the same weight. Anything with the baby's name or birthstone on it, such as jewelry, is also customary. Any of the traditional keepsakes will also work such as something to preserve a lock of hair, handprints/footprints, molds and books or special boxes to keep pictures in.
- Offer to make phone calls for them.

- Send a card. There is actually a line of cards for pregnancy and infant loss by Hallmark and other card makers.
- Be comfortable in their tears.
- Attend the funeral/memorial service.
- Send a daily message but do not expect a response. "How are you today?" "Thinking of you." "Hope things are going okay."
- Understand that the next year will be a "year of firsts." Going into their home without their baby will be a "first," returning to work will be a "first," going to the same grocery store will be a "first," and any holiday will be a "first" holiday without their baby. There will be many "firsts."
- Remember the baby's birthday/angel date/death date. Send a card, make a phone call, send a text. It can be as simple as "Remembering your baby's (can insert baby's name) birth today."
- Remember the baby's due date – If their baby died before their due date, this will be a particularly difficult day. Let them know you are thinking of them and you are there.
- Be supportive in the weeks and months to come.
- Attend memorial events – Be there for the funeral or any memorial events and find local walks and other annual remembrance events to help them share their baby.
- Set up a meal train/calendar of people who will bring them meals. Soups can be hearty and healthy. Bringing veggie trays, fruit trays, sandwich trays, or just setting out some healthy food can be extremely helpful. It is a

reminder that the family needs to eat, which is often put on hold while mourning.

- Bring household items such as milk, eggs, butter, toilet paper, paper towels, paper plates, aluminum foil, toothpaste, etc.
- Mow the lawn, take out the trash, bring in the trash cans, etc.
- Pick up around the house (do laundry, mow the lawn, empty and load the dishwasher, make the beds, etc). Do not break down the baby's nursery or remove any items for the baby.

Chapter Thirteen:
Veterans

This section was written by Tamara Wedin, Founder of Taps for Babies

Veteran Families

If you or your partner are military veterans, you may be navigating your healthcare within the Veterans Health Administration. This gives you access to a lot of resources, but it may be difficult to search them out while grieving. Here's a list of services you can ask about, whether you are already using the VA or not. Some services will require enrolling in VA, and others are available to all veterans.

Chaplain Services

Chaplain Services are available for all veterans, regardless of era or whether or not they are already enrolled in the VA. You can call the main VA hospital switchboard and ask to be connected to Chaplain Services, and request an appointment to speak with a Chaplain. As with active duty

Chaplains, VA Chaplains are trained to help people across many belief systems, including those who don't have a strong leaning towards any belief. Chaplain Services also has knowledge of programs you can ask about, such as Warrior to Soulmate, which is a program that helps couples to grow in communication together. These can be helpful after a loss. Grief support groups are also often offered through Chaplain Services, though these groups will sometimes encompass many different types of grief together. All of these services are free.

Women's Clinic

Women Veterans who are eligible for VA services are eligible to have their prenatal and maternity care (including delivery and first seven days of baby's life) covered through VA. For those who were not using this coverage, you can still inquire about supportive services following a miscarriage. The best person to speak with would be the Women Veteran Program Manager. VA is just beginning to really understand and implement support after a miscarriage, and there may or may not be anything already in place, but it is worth asking about.

Mental Health Services

Many more veterans are eligible for services from the Mental Health clinic than know it. Contrary to popular belief, issues you are seen for do not have to revolve around service. Couples can receive family counseling or grief counseling together, even if both are not veterans. Counseling can also be done alone for the veteran. It is important to recognize what support you may be needing before things get too overwhelming. While miscarriage itself can cause post-traumatic stress, a loss can also trigger previous trauma and make symptoms previously managed, less managed. Often in military culture there is a perception that asking for mental health help is a sign of weakness, but the opposite is true. It requires a lot of strength to ask for help and to do the hard work that comes with managing trauma. Mental Health referrals happen a variety of ways. They can come through a primary care provider, from a VA urgent care or VA emergency room visit, or Chaplain Services. Some VAs also have a Mental Health triage clinic, where you can be seen the same day for urgent matters.

Other VA programs

Some VA facilities offer programs that cannot be found in every VA, for example: trauma-sensitive yoga, Healing Touch, or acupuncture. Several VAs also have art therapy or community partnerships where different forms of art (painting, collage, photography, writing) are being explored with groups of veterans or community members as a way to express what's going on inside. This can be very healing. If doing this in a group of others who understand military and veteran culture, and the gut response to "keep on keepin' on" would be helpful, ask around at the VA departments listed above, as well as with VA Voluntary Services (the main switchboard can get you to them), who may be aware of local projects going on. Your eligibility for some of these programs will vary, especially if the partner having the miscarriage is not the veteran, and in some cases, a referral from a primary care provider in VA will be required, however, many of these types of programs are sponsored by community partners and are eligible to any veteran who wishes to participate.

National Cemetery Administration

National Cemetery Administration has a burial benefit for most veterans who lose a dependent child. When dealing with a loss before birth, it is best to check with the National Cemetery in your area to find out what burial or cremation options you may be eligible for. Many veterans have had their miscarried babies buried for free at a National Cemetery, where headstone and care are included. They may also be able to suggest funeral homes who have compassionate rates for babies, if these are options you want to look into.

The Vet Center

If you are a combat veteran or veterans who has experienced military sexual trauma (MST), you can take your DD214 in to a Vet Center with no appointment. These centers offer free counseling regardless of eligibility for VA services. The MST does not need to be noted in your record. They also offer bereavement support to those who have lost a service member, and you may be able to inquire about seeing one of these counselors if you feel that your miscarriage is causing any additional stress to any service-related combat stress or stress from your MST. Often these counselors will come to the home.

Taps for Babies

Taps for Babies is a non-profit that provides advocacy, support and resource referrals for veteran and military families who experience pregnancy loss, infant loss, or fertility issues. Visit TapsForBabies.org to learn more, find their Facebook page, as well as a closed peer support group just for the military and veteran families who have had the loss. If you need any assistance tracking down specific resources in your community or VA, or if you would like to connect to veteran or military peer support after a miscarriage, Taps for Babies can help with that.

Make the Connection

Make the Connection is an online VA program that offers a variety of tools for veterans to track down support that works for them. Online self-assessments, connections to stories of other veterans who have gone through similar challenges, and is a great place to find out about other programs that can help you to focus on self-care while healing from your miscarriage. Notable programs include MOVE! (a free weight management program), Moving Forward (a multiple step program for managing stress during difficult times and overcoming challenging life events, a free app is also available), Parenting2Go (a parenting program that helps parents of living children to manage stress in parenting and to redirect and focus on family-healthy techniques for working through issues, a free app is also available), and PTSD Coach Online (an award-winning program to assist veterans in managing trauma through modules and coaching online). These programs are available to all veteran families at no cost.

Team Red, White and Blue

Often veterans find comfort in being with other veterans while sorting out issues, so becoming involved with a group that understands a different way of processing grief can provide your family support, even without it being grief specific. Many are aware of their local American Legion, or Veterans of Foreign Wars posts, but another to look for is Team Red, White and Blue. Team RWB's mission is to "enrich the lives of America's veterans by connecting them to their community through physical and social activity." You do not need to be a veteran to join, it is family-friendly, and Facebook groups keep members connected to a strong sense of team. Physical activity can be especially helpful during the grief process.

Coaching Into Care

For those who love and care for veterans who may need additional support, Coaching Into Care has counselors and psychologists available Monday through Friday, 8 am to 8 pm (ET) to provide guidance, tips and help for connecting your veteran to help inside the VA. Their number is 888-823-7458.

Chapter Fourteen: Other Resources

Books for Her

All That is Seen and Unseen; A Journey Through a First Trimester Miscarriage by Elizabeth Petrucelli

Miscarriage: Women Sharing From the Heart by Marie Allen

Empty Arms: Coping With Miscarriage, Stillbirth and Infant Death by Sherokee Ilse

After Miscarriage: A Catholic Woman's Companion to Healing & Hope by Karen Edmisten

I Never Held You: Miscarriage, Grief, Healing and Recovery by Ellen M. DuBois

Books for Him

Father in Crisis: The Invisible Child by Burt Wilber

A Guide for Father's When a Baby Dies by Tim Nelson

Books for Children

Something Happened: A book for children and parents who have experienced pregnancy loss by Cathy Blanford

Someone Came Before You by Pat Schwiebert

Books for Grandparents

A Grandparent's Sorrow by Pat Schwiebert

For Bereaved Grandparents by Margaret Gerner

Songs

Bring the Rain by Mercy Me

Gone Too Soon by Daughtry

Held by Natalie Grant

I Will Carry You by Selah

Precious Child by Karen Taylor Good

Support

HEALing Embrace

Nationalshare.org

Stillmothers.com (living childless after loss)

The Miscarriage Association (US) and (UK)

Chapter Fifteen:
Tear-outs

These are extra pages for you to tear out and hand to others or utilize on your healing journey.

What to Say

"I don't know what to say."

"Who can I call for you?" (Be prepared to actually make those phone calls).

"Be patient with yourself. Grief has no timeline."

"Don't feel guilty because you laughed today."

"Can I take your baby's siblings to the park? I know you don't feel like laughing or playing right now."

"I am going to the store, can I bring anything back for you?"

"Talk to me. I am here to listen."

"I am out running errands, is there anything you need?"

"How are you doing today?"

"You don't have to answer the phone or call me back, I just wanted to check in on you."

"How about I take your baby's siblings to school, or grandma's, or ____?"

"I would love to attend a support group with you or go to church with you."

What Not to Say

"You can have another baby."

"At least you know you can get pregnant."

"It was God's way of protecting you from ____."

"It was God's will."

"Heaven needed another angel."

"Your baby is better in Heaven."

"Time heals all wounds."

"I know just how you feel." (Unless you have personally experienced pregnancy loss).

"It could have been worse."

"Now you have an angel/saint in Heaven."

"You should be over this by now! It's been ____ weeks/months/years."

"God never gives us more than we can handle."

"What can I do for you?" Instead say, "Can I do ___ for you? Or "I am going to bring over a meal" not "Can I bring over a meal?"

Things You Can Do

- Listen – They may want to talk over and over again about the pregnancy and the death experience. Be the person they can go to and vent with and repeat their story. Most people want to stop listening after the 3rd or 4th time.
- Bring tissues.
- Give them a hug.
- Encourage the family to have pictures taken with their baby.
- Ask and hold the baby.
- Be their shoulder to cry on. If they don't want to talk, they may just want someone to lean on while they cry. Let them cry. Crying is just one way to express grief.
- Cry with them. You don't have to be stoic. Crying helps validate that this is a sad time and an experience worth grieving. They will not be angry with you for crying.
- Be there – For the birth that is. If you would have most likely been there for the birth anyway, be sure to let them know you would still like to be there to support them. At the very least, the family may prefer you wait in the waiting room (which can be typical at a live birth too).
- Call their baby by name – which may seem weird. Unless the family does not want you to call their baby by name, this is preferred.
- Mementos – Bring something for them to remember their baby by. For any birth, people give gifts. This is no different although the gifts might be slightly different. The family may want an outfit, so ask. Families are often encouraged to dress their baby just like they

would at a live birth. A teddy bear that is at least 14 inches but less than 24 inches is best as well. Mom can hold the bear as she leaves the hospital. You can also find out the baby's weight and make a bear of the same weight. Anything with the baby's name or birthstone on it, such as jewelry, is also customary. Any of the traditional keepsakes will also work such as something to preserve a lock of hair, handprints/footprints, molds and books or special boxes to keep pictures in.

- Offer to make phone calls for them.
- Send a card. There is actually a line of cards for pregnancy and infant loss by Hallmark and other card makers.
- Be comfortable in their tears.
- Attend the funeral/memorial service.
- Send a daily message but do not expect a response. "How are you today?" "Thinking of you." "Hope things are going okay."
- Understand that the next year will be a "year of firsts." Going into their home without their baby will be a "first," returning to work will be a "first," going to the same grocery store will be a "first," and any holiday will be a "first" holiday without their baby. There will be many "firsts."
- Remember the baby's birthday/angel date/death date. Send a card, make a phone call, send a text. It can be as simple as "Remembering your baby's (can insert baby's name) birth today."
- Remember the baby's due date – If their baby died before their due date, this will be a particularly difficult day. Let them know you are thinking of them and you are there.

- Be supportive in the weeks and months to come.
- Attend memorial events – Be there for the funeral or any memorial events and find local walks and other annual remembrance events to help them share their baby.
- Set up a meal train/calendar of people who will bring them meals. Soups can be hearty and healthy. Bringing veggie trays, fruit trays, sandwich trays, or just setting out some healthy food can be extremely helpful. It is a reminder that the family needs to eat, which is often put on hold while mourning.
- Bring household items such as milk, eggs, butter, toilet paper, paper towels, paper plates, aluminum foil, toothpaste, etc.
- Mow the lawn, take out the trash, bring in the trash cans, etc.

Pick up around the house (do laundry, mow the lawn, empty and load the dishwasher, make the beds, etc). Do not break down the baby's nursery or remove any items for the baby.

Going Back to Work

Scripted message to co-workers. (Adapt to your needs)

On March 18th, I learned I was expecting baby #2. My husband and I had been trying for another baby for about three years. We were very excited and began preparing for this baby, but on April 14th, we learned the baby no longer had a heartbeat. We were devastated and our six-year-old son was crushed. It has been very hard on all of us and I am still very sad about this loss. Although it has been two weeks since we had our baby, I find myself crying from time to time for no reason. We do not know the reason for our loss and would appreciate your support as we navigate through our grief.

I understand that this can be uncomfortable for some people and everyone has different beliefs so I have included a list of what to say and what not to say that many find helpful. In addition, we named our baby Ruby and would love for you to address our baby by her name.

What to Say

"I don't know what to say."
"Be patient with yourself. Grief has no timeline."
"Don't feel guilty because you laughed today."
"I am going to the store, can I bring anything back for you?"
"Talk to me. I am here to listen."
"I am out running errands, is there anything you need?"
"How are you doing today?"

"You don't have to answer the phone or call me back, I just wanted to check in on you."
"I would love to attend a support group with you or go to church with you."

What Not to Say

"You can have another baby."
"At least you know you can get pregnant."
"It was God's way of protecting you from ____."
"It was God's will."
"Heaven needed another angel."
"Your baby is better in Heaven."
"Time heals all wounds."
"I know just how you feel." (Unless you have personally experienced pregnancy loss).
"It could have been worse."
"You should be over this by now! It's been ____ weeks/months/years."
"God never gives us more than we can handle."
"What can I do for you?" Instead say, "Can I do ___ for you? Or "I am going to bring over a meal" not "Can I bring over a meal?"

Going Out in Public

Scripted message to those in public. (Adapt to your needs)

I was expecting a baby, but my baby died. I cannot speak the words. Please do not offer reasons for my baby's death or try to put a positive spin on this. Thank you for understanding.

Healthy Ways to Grieve

- Join a support group (if none exist, start one)
- Journal (daily, weekly, monthly)
- Art (drawing, making pottery)
- Crafts (making miscarriage bracelets, burial gowns, burial boxes, baby blankets)
- Write a letter to your baby
- Write a letter to you from your baby
- Write a letter to God
- Get a bear or stuffed animal that weighs the same as your baby did
- Publish your story (online, in a blog, in a book, in a magazine)
- Become a bereavement doula
- Stay away from drugs, alcohol and smoking.

Caring for Your Postpartum Body

- Take naps and try to get plenty of rest.
- Limit visitors unless visits are emotionally healing for you.
- Watch your bleeding.
- If you begin to bleed heavily, you did too much.
- Nothing in your vagina for six weeks.
- Restrict lifting (items less than 15 pounds).
- Household chores should be put on hold or completed by someone else for the first few weeks while your body heals.
- Eat healthy foods.
- Drink plenty of fluids (at least six to eight glasses of water per day)
- Change your pads every two to three hours.
- Use your peribottle (if you received one).
- A hemorrhoid pillow can help with vaginal pain experienced while sitting/getting up from sitting.
- Increase your fiber intake.
- Take short walks every day.
- Urinate every three to five hours.
- Do not drive if you are taking any narcotics for pain.
- Avoid smoking, illegal drugs, alcohol and limit caffeine consumption.

Collecting and Storing Breast Milk

Collecting

- Wash your hands thoroughly.
- Pump or express directly into a collection bag or bottle.

Sterilizing Pump Parts

Be sure to clean your pump parts after each pump. There are a few ways to do this.

- Use PURE IVORY soap and a brush and clean the parts in warm soapy water making sure to clean all the membranes and corners of the connectors. Air dry.
- Use the Medela Steam bags. Rinse the parts and follow the directions on the steam bag. Make sure you do this directly after pumping so no milk has a chance to dry on the parts.
- For when you are on the go, use Medela Anti-bacterial wipes to clean your parts. You do not have to rinse with water, but it won't hurt.
- For an exclusive pumper, you may pump and then seal your parts in a bag (without rinsing) and place in the refrigerator. Clean your parts using one of the methods above at the end of each day.

Storage

There are many items on the market for storing breast milk. If you are storing for short periods of time, use a plastic or glass container. When filling the bottle, be sure to leave a little space at the top. Breast milk is made of water and will expand and break your bottles rendering your milk useless. Label the container with the date and amount.

If you will be storing long term, use bags as they take up less freezer space. Lansinoh Breastmilk Storage bags freeze flat and take up less room in a freezer. Label the bag with the date and amount. It's okay to use a black marker, it will not seep into the milk.

- Store the milk in the coldest section of the freezer. Do not allow the bag or bottle to touch the sides of a self-defrosting freezer! These types of freezers prevent frost by warming the sides, thus warming your milk.
- Freeze milk within four to six days.
- Freezing amounts of two ounces works well for the first few months.

Layering Milk

You may add fresh milk to previously pumped refrigerated milk. It is recommended that you cool the milk before mixing it with the already cooled milk. Never add warm milk to frozen milk.

Daily Tasks

When someone asks, "How can I help?" many times the response is "I don't know," or the family struggles to communicate their needs. Use the chart on the following page to list your daily tasks.

Place the chart on your refrigerator or in another conspicuous place. When the question "How can I help?" or "Is there anything I can do for you?" is asked, you can refer them to the chart.

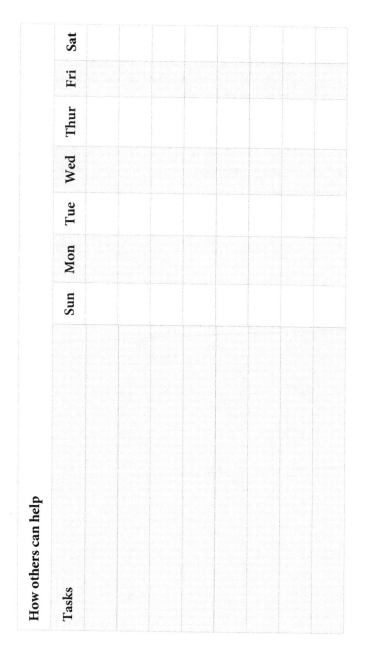

Tasks	How others can help	Sun	Mon	Tue	Wed	Thur	Fri	Sat

Bibliography

1.   "Miscarriage: MedlinePlus Medical Encyclopedia."
U.S National Library of Medicine. U.S. National Library of
Medicine, Web. 16 Jan. 2015.
http://www.nlm.nih.gov/medlineplus/ency/article/001488.
htm

2.   "Evaluation of Fetal Death." Evaluation of Fetal
Death. Web. 16 Jan. 2015.
http://emedicine.medscape.com/article/259165-overview

3.   "Miscarriage - American Pregnancy Association."
American Pregnancy Association Miscarriage Comments,
26 Apr. 2012. Web. 16 Jan. 2015.
http://americanpregnancy.org/pregnancy-
complications/miscarriage/

4.   "Molar Pregnancy - American Pregnancy
Association." American Pregnancy Association. 26 Apr.
2012. Web. 17 Jan. 2015.
http://americanpregnancy.org/pregnancy-
complications/molar-pregnancy/

5.   Blum, J., B. Winikoff, K. Gemzell-Danielsson, P.C.
Ho, R. Schiavon, and A. Weeks. "Treatment of Incomplete
Abortion and Miscarriage with Misoprostal." International
Journal of Gynecology and Obsetrics 99 (2007): S186--189.
Web.
http://www.misoprostol.org/File/IJGO_incomp_Blum.pdf

6.   "How Many People Are Affected by or at Risk for Pregnancy Loss or Miscarriage?" National Institute of Child Health and Development 30 Nov. 2012. Web. 17 Jan. 2015.
http://www.nichd.nih.gov/health/topics/pregnancyloss/con ditioninfo/Pages/risk.aspx

7.   National Center for Biotechnology Information. U.S. National Library of Medicine, Web. 17 Jan. 2015.
http://www.ncbi.nlm.nih.gov/pubmed/18310375

8.   "Second Trimester Pregnancy Loss." - American Family Physician. Web. 17 Jan. 2015.
http://www.aafp.org/afp/2007/1101/p1341.html

OTHER BOOKS BY ELIZABETH PETRUCELLI

All That is Seen and Unseen; A Journey Through a First Trimester Miscarriage

facebook.com/allthatisseenandunseen
Follow her blog at allthatisseenandunseen.com

The First Night; Small Town Fumblings of a Rookie Police Officer

facebook.com/TheFirstNightBook

Visit elizabethpetrucelli.com for more upcoming books!